BELLY FAT
40 EFFECTIVE HABITS
TO BURN BELLY FAT
FOR A SLIM WAIST

I0414102

TIERRA RUBIO

BOOK DESCRIPTION

Are you having a hard time losing that belly fat?

Belly fat is not attractive, let us face that fact. Most people would kill for a well chiseled and athletic body. Belly fat may also contribute to the development of various health complications like diabetes.

If you are struggling to get rid of that belly fat, then this book is for you!

This book aims to provide the most effective ways to lose belly fat. I am going to share with you the easy-to-follow effective habits that will make losing belly fat look an easy task. I will explain the factors that contribute to belly fat and how you can keep the belly fat from growing.

You will get to know how your eating habits have been the cause of the belly fat. You will pick up the right eating habits to adapt to keep belly fat at bay. I will also share with you the working out habits and how they contribute to belly fat loss. You will learn the most effective workout exercises in losing belly fat. I will also talk about the lifestyle you choose to lead and its impact in making you have belly fat. You will learn to live to avoid belly fat and have a leaner and healthier body. This book aims at showing you the root causes of belly fat and how you can eliminate it.

This is THE BOOK to help YOU lose that belly fat once and for all.

Table of Contents

INTRODUCTION

Belly fat is a menace to most people, who have run out of ideas on how to get rid of it. However belly fat is mainly a result of the habits you employ in your life. Losing belly fat is not hard but maintaining the flat belly is the most difficult part. Most people have shed belly fat unknowingly maybe as a result of a strenuous activity or not affording fast foods. The belly fat loss may have been superficial but if you are able to adjust your life habits to ones that enable you to lose the belly fat and stick to these habits, you will definitely have a flat belly and finally have a sight of your abs.

The habits that you should watch out for are eating, workout and lifestyle habits. These habits are the real reason behind the increase in belly fat cases. You can't change one or two of these habits, but all of the three to get the results you are looking for.

Here's what you will learn:

17 Eating Habits

The eating habits are the habits that make the way for belly fat to accumulate. You should watch what you eat and how it is beneficial to your health. The best way to adjust to healthy eating habits is to reflect on the bad eating habits you were used to and replace them with good and healthy eating habits. Changing to healthy eating habits may prove difficult because old habits die hard. You have to keep on reinforcing the healthy eating habits until they become a part of you.

15 Workout Habits

Workout habits don't just help you lose the belly fat but help you maintain and stay in shape. The best works out habits are those that aim the abdominal core, where the belly fat accumulates and hardens the core making you more lean and muscular. Thus to achieve effective belly fat lose, you have to do exercises that target the belly area and ensure that you shed as much fat as possible around the area. Make it a habit to always work out because the belly fat can easily creep back if you neglect your well-being by failing to hit the gym and exercise.

8 Lifestyle Habits

Lifestyle habits are serial and silent habits that make the belly fat accumulate and you have no idea how it happened. Following the right kind of lifestyle habits will get you on the right track and it will give you the sense of successes in gradually getting rid of that belly fat. Even after getting in shape, you will never have to worry about the belly fat reoccurring because these lifestyle habits work in a natural and automatic way.

This book aims at providing the 40 effective habits based on the main three habits, that is, eating, workout and lifestyle habits. The habits get rid of that belly fat and keep it away.

BASICS OF BELLY FAT

The human skin has a layer of fat underneath it called subcutaneous fat. The subcutaneous fat makes about 80 percent to 90 percent of the total body fat. It is normally found on the back of the arms, below the shoulder blades, around the belly and on the upper legs and hips. The remaining 20 to 10 percent of the total body fat is located below the stomach muscles and around other internal organs such as the kidneys, spleen, livers and intestines. This 20 percent to 10 percent body fat is referred to as belly fat.

The subcutaneous fat layer has two main functions in the body. These functions are keeping your body warm and acting as storage for certain hormones and body energy. The subcutaneous fat is very helpful especially in cases of famine when other energy sources, carbohydrates and proteins are not available. It becomes a readily available source of energy keeping the cell metabolism going. On acting as an endocrine organ, the subcutaneous fat layer contains numerous hormones. The leptin hormone, for example, which relays to the brain that you have had enough to eat is located in this fat layer.

Belly fat is very different from the subcutaneous fat; in fact, it is more harmful. Belly fat has been found to increase the risk factors of type 2 diabetes, cardiovascular and inflammatory diseases. The reason why your belly protrudes outwards is that the belly fat is much firmer than the subcutaneous fat and thus pushes your abdominal muscles outwards and accumulates around the abdominal core. The fat cells located deep in the abdomen, do not release free fatty acids into the bloodstream instead their fatty acids are transported to the liver. The liver, in turn, changes the fatty acids to other forms of fats, that is, triglyceride and cholesterol. These forms of fats are then secreted into the bloodstream. When the fat cell is broken down and transported in the blood, the broken down form is referred to as free fatty acid which is utilized by the body to produce energy. The triglyceride fat is not harmful as it is also found in the bloodstream and can easily be converted to energy. However, when the levels of the triglyceride and cholesterol are high, you are at high risk of developing a cardiovascular complication.

The accumulation of belly fat has been linked to having low levels of fat burning hormones, high levels of fat storing hormones, sedentary lifestyle, genetic factors. Other minor factors include age and eating too much-processed foods. The reasons for belly fat are related to the habits we take up. These habits will be discussed in this book and effective ways on how to go about them are provided.

PART 1:
EATING HABITS

Eating habits are the precursors of belly fat accumulation. You should watch what you eat in terms of the calorific value of the food and the type of fat in the food. Ensure that the food you take is low in saturated Trans fat and high in monosaturated or unsaturated fats. Unsaturated fats are easily broken down by the body and used to produce energy in the absence of carbohydrates and protein. Your eating habits should be based on the concept of cutting down calorie intake and burning belly fat. The following are some of the healthy eating habits that will help you lose belly fat:

EATING HABIT 1: Change to Healthy Cooking Methods

Losing belly fat will require you to change your cooking methods to healthier ones. Your belly fat may be as a result of using cooking methods that make you eat too many calories in terms of the spices, cooking fat and choice of recipe. Some cooking methods also deplete the nutrients in the foods that are supposed to play a major role in helping you lose the belly fat. It is important during cooking that you ensure that the food is well cooked with no need of additional additives on the table. Most food additives are also directly associated with gaining fat, especially around the belly. When you are consuming vegetables, you should not let them overcook, as this makes them lose their nutrients and hence do not help your body in any way.

EATING HABIT 2: Eat Healthy Portion Sizes

Consuming a little more than you should is the reason why you have a big belly with too much fat in it. The body requires a small percentage of what we eat for its optimal cell metabolism. The rest of the food ingredient is eliminated as waste or stored as fat for later energy use. The more food you eat makes you consume too many calories and sugars. The excess sugars are converted and stored in the body as fat especially around the belly.

You are just supposed to eat a small portion of food with all the essential nutrients for your body growth and development. You should avoid taking large food portions rather divide your meals so that you can have small portions of food a maximum of five days a day. The mentality of having three meals a day is also misleading and encourages belly fat accumulation. This is because the three meals a day principle makes you overeat during meal time and as a result, you exceed your healthy daily calorie intake. It is important that you cut your meal proportions to smaller sizes and instead have healthy snacks in between the breakfast, lunch and dinner meals. This helps you to consume less and you never get hungry and so have your cravings in check. You can choose to have fruits as your snacks or healthier processed foods like chocolates and chips, but make sure the foods are low in calories and within the allowed daily calorie. This helps you to lose belly fat and also enables you to maintain the flat belly when you achieve it.

EATING HABIT 3: Keep A Food Log

A good healthy eating habit that will help you lose the belly fat includes having a food log where you state every food you eat. This ensures that you keep tabs of a number of calories you are consuming with every food item. A food log will help you be able to avoid foods that are high in calories and likely to encourage the accumulation of belly fat. Writing down the foods you are having helps you come up with a healthy and effective diet plan that will help you lose the belly fat and get in shape with time. Most people fail in losing the belly fat because they do not note down the food they take and in the long run end up consuming more calories which consequently makes them add fat, especially around the abdominal area.

EATING HABIT 4: Plan Your Healthy Shopping: Food To Look For And Food To Avoid

Losing belly fat means changing what you usually buy from the food stores and going for healthier alternatives. You should stock your fridge with fruits and vegetables that are healthier for you and your family. You should build a home cooking culture in your home and when the fridge and shelves do not have food supplies, this will encourage you to buy junk food so that you do not have to cook and just sit around and watch TV. Always make sure that you get healthy supplies from the store on your way from work. This helps you have full control of the diet process and ensure that you are eating and losing the belly fat every day.

FOOD TO LOOK FOR

The following are the best foods, mainly fruits and vegetables to go for when shopping and which will actually help in burning the belly fat:

1) Walnuts

Among all nuts, walnuts are the best when you are losing belly fat. Walnuts contain twice the antioxidants found in other nuts. It is an amazing weight management food which also helps lower the cholesterol levels in the body. However, as much as walnuts help in weight loss, they are high in calories and should be consumed in moderation. You should consider taking walnuts as part of your snacks when you are resting.

2) Almonds

Almonds are good weight management foods. They are also full of nutrients including folic acid, vitamin E, monosaturated fats, protein and fibre. The almonds help keep the blood sugar constant, making you feel full and avoid overeating. The almonds can be served with bread during breakfast or taken as snacks when passing time or while on the road. If you happen to consume an unhealthy food, you can follow up with some almonds. The almonds help the body to maintain optimal blood sugar and prevent the formation of excess fat from the digestion of the unhealthy food eaten.

3) Bananas

Bananas should also be included in your belly loss diet. This is because they contain the mineral potassium, which is responsible for lowering blood pressure. It also contains Tryptophan, which has been found to help reduce depression. Bananas are also high in iron mineral which helps in preventing anaemia and lowers irregular bowel movements. The main reason a banana is incorporated in a belly loss diet is that it contains high protein and soluble fibre, which makes it ideal to stabilize blood sugar. Stabilizing of blood sugar prevents the rise in insulin which may is responsible for the formation of excess fats mainly around the abdominal area.

4) Tomatoes

It has been found that the consumption of a tomato prompts the body to release a hormone, cholecystokinin, which makes you feel full and satisfied. This is advantageous as it helps you to avoid overeating. This keeps your cravings at bay helping you not to add any excess calories or fats around the abdominal area.

Another plus is that tomatoes are very low in calories making them ideal in avoiding adding excess fat. Tomatoes also help maintain normal blood sugar and minimize cholesterol in the body.

5) Spinach

Spinach is a very good vegetable when it comes to losing fat in the body. It contains vitamins A, K, fibre, antioxidants, magnesium potassium and iron. It has low calorific value and a serving of its juice or as a vegetable will make you feel full and suppress your cravings and help you avoid overeating.

6) Apples

An apple a day keeps the doctor away, so it is said. There is almost nothing an apple can't fix in the body including fat loss. The Apple is very low in calories making it a good food to consume when on a belly loss diet. The Apple is also rich in fibre which makes you feel full for a longer time as it takes more time to break down the fibre.

7) Lentils

Lentils are effective belly flatteners. They contain high protein content and fibre material. This makes them help the body be able to maintain the body sugar at normal levels. Normal blood sugar prevents the abnormal rise of insulin in the body which results to the body creating excess fats, especially around the abdominal areas. Lentils are prepared easily, so in case you are tired and not in the mood for cooking a large meal in accordance with your diet plan, you can just resort to cooking lentils which will cook fast and in a short time.

8) Beetroot

Drinking beetroot juice will give you a burst of energy. This gives the body the ability to endure and last longer when carrying out rigorous workout exercises. This enables you to burn more calories and loses considerable amount of belly fat with time. So next time you hit the gym, carry some beetroot juice with you.

Beetroot is also a natural blood detoxifier and replenishes it with minerals and natural sugars. Beetroot is rich in beta-carotene, vitamins A, C, calcium and fibre material.

9) Black Beans

Beans remain in your digestive system longer and also include in the sensation of fullness with a satisfied feeling, assisting fat burning. They consist of soluble with insoluble fibre, healthy protein, with a kind of fat-burning carbohydrate called resistant starch. Black beans are actually one of the greatest fat burning foods. Bean eaters weigh much less with have slimmer middles.

They are a 'heart healthy and balanced' addition to any sort of diet regimen as they include a wealth of soluble fibre, which could reduce cholesterol and also triglyceride degrees. This weight loss food is abundant with essential nutrients like monosaturated fats, vitamin E, folic acid, a protein with dietary fibre. This weight loss food additionally keeps your blood sugar constant.

10) Garlic

The garlic is an effective fat burning ingredient. It is zero in calories and it has been found to help people shed a considerable amount of fat in a short period of time. It is sprinkled in the food as a natural additive. It is also a good appetite controller and helps you avoid overeating and promote weight loss.

11) Cabbage

Cabbage is a readily available leafy vegetable no matter the geographical location. This weight loss vegetable is the ideal ingredient to include in your meals as your target to lose the belly fat. It has a low calorific value and high in fibre content which makes you feel full and hence keep your hunger in check for a long time. Cabbage is also high in vitamin C which helps the body fight infections especially lowering the risk factor of diabetes mellitus.

12) Pears

Pears are very high in fibre content which helps you feel full for a longer time after consuming them. The pears are effective in helping to lose the belly fat as they are also low in calories. The pears also help to eliminate free radicals in the body which are also linked to adding weight and fat in the body.

13) Lean Healthy Protein

Lean healthy protein is a good belly fat burning foods with the ability to keep your food cravings in check. Nonvegans can get their lean protein from lean meat, fish and eggs. Vegetarians can resort to getting their protein from tofu, soya beans, chickpeas and peanut butter. Protein promotes fat loss and the more you consume proteins and cut on carbohydrates, you are able to shed considerable fat especially around the belly area.

14) Eggs

Eggs also can play a major role in helping lose belly fat. They are good sources of vitamins, essential minerals and protein. Eggs make you feel satisfied and full and help you avoid overeating and hence help in belly fat loss.

FOOD TO AVOID AND BOOST FAT LOSS

You can effectively lose belly fat by eliminating or restricting intake of specific types of foods that can hinder fat loss. Avoid food made with refined grains (white rice, white bread, and regular pasta) and baked goods. These are really delicious, but they are not worth it. Those packed doughnuts, mini muffins, or chocolate cupcakes will only increase your calorie and sugar intake, and they are also not easy to digest.

You should avoid white flour which contains refined sugars. The refined sugars are quickly digested by the body leading to high insulin and blood sugars levels. The high insulin and blood sugar levels cause fat accumulation and storage around the belly area. Instead, you should replace the white flour with whole-grain flour.

Also avoid salty chips, fried foods, high-fat meat such as pork, and sweet beverages such as sodas, canned fruit juices, lemonade, and sweetened tea. Replace these drinks with plain water, iced water. You can add lemon or herbs to the water to enhance its taste. Drinking a lot of simple sugars through fizzy drinks can lead to spikes in insulin levels. An increase in insulin promotes increased fat storage in the belly area, Choose calorie-free drinks, such as water or unsweetened green tea.

EATING HABIT 5: Make Water Your Primary Drink

Water plays a major role in helping you lose the belly fat. This is because water makes you feel full and minimal calories. This is ideal for cutting your calorie intake. After taking your breakfast, the rest of the day just make water your primary drink. This keeps your cravings in control and ensures that you do not overeat.

Avoid soft drinks which are high in calories due to the added sugars. The added sugars will only come in the way of you and lose the belly fat. Worse, the sugary drinks trigger your cravings and only make you want you to eat. This makes you overeat and hence more calories for your body to turn and store as fats around your belly. So if you really want to make that belly fat disappear, forego sweetened drinks and make water a priority.

EATING HABIT 6: Don't Eliminate Fats From Your Diet

Actually, people think that eliminating fats from their diet will help them lose the belly fat. However, this will only make you put more weight. The thing about fats is that it makes you feel full and helps suppress your food cravings. Fats also help the body absorb various nutrients and fats in the food. So you should not be afraid of including fats in your diet, it will be beneficial in losing the belly fat.

EATING HABIT 7: Don't Skip Breakfast

Skipping breakfast in your diet plan is not a good idea because it has been proven to be an important meal. Breakfast gives you the necessary nutrients and energy you require to tackle your busy day. Breakfast will help you feel full and avoid overeating in the afternoon. The most effective breakfast in losing belly fat is one that is high in fibre and low in sugar and sodium.

Research shows people that do not miss their breakfast are more likely to have a flat belly compared to people who skip breakfast. Breakfast increases cell metabolism and helps you burn more calories throughout the day. If you miss breakfast, your body registers that there is a shortage of nutrients and its reaction is slowing metabolism to make the available nutrients last long. Thus the body is not able to burn more calories when you skip breakfast.

EATING HABIT 8: Take Your Time When Eating

You should develop a habit of not hurrying when you are having your meals. You should develop a diet plan that allows you to have adequate time to eat and that you are never hungry throughout the day. One reason for eating too fast is being super hungry. So avoid putting yourself in a situation where you are feeling so hungry that all you can think of is food. Eating too fast makes you overeat while eating slowly helps you know when it is okay to stop eating and just take a cup of water and you are satisfied.

EATING HABIT 9: Stop Eating All The Food On Your Plate

The childhood thought that you eat all the food on your plate will make you grow even faster is wrong. If you do not get this act under control, it becomes a habit and you end up always clearing everything in the plate. Develop a habit of leaving some food on the table in case the food is a lot. This helps you to keep your calorie intake under control and avoiding adding more weight, especially around the abdominal area.

EATING HABIT 10: Eat Healthy Unprocessed Food

There has been an increase in the consumption of processed and packaged foods over the years. This is a dangerous trend and one of the reasons for the increase in obesity and overweight cases. The problem is that the packaged foods do not contain balanced nutrients. They are high in fat, salt sugar and lack essential nutrients and fibre. You should develop the habit of preparing meals from unprocessed foods which unlike processed foods are high in essential nutrients and fibre. The unprocessed foods are low in calories and have soluble monosaturated fats which are easily broken down by the body. This allows you to be able to shed the excess fat around the belly and with time you will lose the fat and have a flat belly and better still realize that you were also born with a six pack abs.

EATING HABIT 11: Add Fiber To Eliminate Fat

Fibre helps your body to feel full even with few calories, which is beneficial for belly fat loss. It is ideal to include in your diet with non-starchy vegetables including broccoli, fresh peppers, tomatoes, cucumbers, celery, cauliflower, mushrooms, and other leafy greens. It is also recommended to include fruits with low caloric content such as strawberries, melons, and apples. Also eat legumes, nuts and seeds that are rich in protein and in fibre. Choose whole grain bread, cereals, quinoa, and brown rice. These foods are very effective in losing the belly fat and staying fit.

EATING HABIT 12: Increase Oatmeal Consumption

Oatmeal is very rich in fibre, vitamins and minerals, and complex carbohydrates. You can eat plain, unsweetened oatmeal in the morning. To enhance taste, you can add fruits such as banana, strawberries or kiwi. You can also add oats to fruit smoothies for added energy and to control your hunger. Oatmeal will help you stay satisfied and avoid any overeating and thus enabling to lose the belly fat.

EATING HABIT 13: Choose The Right Protein Intake

Choose foods that are rich in protein, which includes dairy products. Based on research, diet plans that are calorie restricted combined with high protein diet and resistance training lead to more belly fat loss compared to a program with a low-protein diet. Be sure to include protein-rich meats such as poultry, egg whites, and seafood.

Red meat such as beef and lamb are the best sources of protein. You should choose the leanest cuts, and get rid of visible fat. Aside from protein, red meat is also a good source of iron, folate, essential fatty acids, and Vitamin B12. Be sure not to overcook red meat to preserve the protein.

It is advisable to serve lean meat during dieting which helps lower the LDL ("bad") cholesterol levels which increase the risk factor of heart diseases. When the protein intake is high than carbohydrates, it promotes ketosis. The body utilizes the stored fats especially belly fat for energy instead of carbohydrates. This makes the body burn fats resulting in fat loss. Ketosis also results to low appetite causing people to eat less food.

Low-fat dairy products are also recommended such as cottage cheese, milk, and plain Greek yoghurt. Aside from protein, these are very rich in calcium that does not only help you build strong and healthy bones, they can also help you to stay fit. Calcium signals the body to absorb less fat regulates blood pressure and helps the body to prevent the onset of osteoporosis. Thus the calcium in the dairy products helps to lower the absorption and storage of fats in the body and hence fewer fats are stored around the belly fat.

Fish is also an important source of protein. Apart from being the richest in protein, fish is also a source of the long-chain omega-3 fatty acids which have a considerable nutritional value. Some of the proven benefits of omega-3 fatty acids that help with belly fat loss include reduction in LDL ("bad") cholesterol, slightly lower blood pressure, reduction in triglycerides, reduce insulin resistance

EATING HABIT 14: Make Nuts Your Friends

Nuts are one of the best foods to help you lose belly fat. This is because they are high in protein, fibre and unsaturated fats. These components play a major role in the body losing excess fats in the body. You should develop a habit of taking nuts as snacks instead of resorting to unhealthy alternatives. So in your dieting make nuts your main foods when you are far from home or not in a position to prepare any healthy recipe.

EATING HABIT 15: Add Low-Salt With Low-Starch Foods In Your Diet

Adding foods low in salt and starch in your diet will help you lose considerable belly fat. Cutting on foods rich in sodium, starch and bad carbohydrates is a very effective way of losing belly fat and can actually result to a permanent flat belly. This is the reason most of the weight loss diets encourage consumption of low salt and low salt foods. Consuming the foods low in sugars and salt significantly cuts your calorie intake and you lose weight and shed fat very quickly.

EATING HABIT 16: Increase Daily Consumption Of Fruits And Vegetables

Most people have embraced the thought that eating from fast foods stores and ordering food to be brought to their doorstep as the right way. This is very wrong and is the main reason for the rise in overweight and obesity across the globe. There has also been immense consumption of processed foods in many homes starting from cornflakes during breakfast to sushi at dinner time. These foods are very dangerous and result in accumulation of unwanted fat in the body especially around the abdominal area. The processed and fast foods are not well balanced in terms of essential nutrients as compared to fruits and vegetables. In fact, they are packed with excess calories that are harmful to the general body health and worse make you add unnecessary weight.

The best solution is to adopt a lifestyle of having fruits and vegetables as much as you can in each meal of the day. The fruits and vegetables are of great value to your body health and weight. You have witnessed how healthy vegans are in terms of weight. This is because the fruits and vegetables contain essential ingredients that are easily broken down and absorbed by the body enzymes. In fact, some of the components in fruits and vegetables replenish the body cells and ensure that they work at their optimal. On the other hand, the fast and processed foods are full of unbalanced ingredients with a proportion of them being harmful to the body cells. These foods are full of fats and calories that make you add necessary weight and some of the harmful ingredients like bad LHL cholesterol result to heart problems and cancer development.

So, in case you are struggling with the belly fat and you haven't shade any considerable weight, drop the fries, hamburgers, pizzas and consider taking fresh fruits and vegetables for a period of at least four months. You will shed that belly fat and in no time you will be able to fully grasp the benefits of fruits and vegetables in having a healthy life and a flat belly. This doesn't mean you have to be so hard on yourself by not having a bite of your favorite foods; you can indeed have a taste by setting aside a single day of the week to have your cakes and chocolates.

EATING HABIT 17: Avoid Binge Drinking

Most people choose to engage in merrymaking and relieving emotional stress by drinking alcohol. Too much alcohol is one of the reasons of having belly fat. This is because alcohol takes precedence and is broken down before any other food you have consumed. This makes the other foods apart from alcohol be stored as fat in the body. Thus, it is important that you avoid binge drinking as it will only make you gain more fat, especially around the belly. For those who love beer should take lighter beers which are low in calories and hence avoid adding unnecessary fats in the body.

So, to lose that belly fat change your lifestyle to one where you do not drink too much alcohol. This lifestyle will ensure that you are able to not only achieve a flat belly but also you can maintain it.

PART 2:
WORKOUT HABITS

Workout habits are hard to develop due to the busy daily work schedule. However, it is important that you create time for you to exercise and burn the belly fat. Workout habits will help you get the lean and healthy body that you wish for. The following are some of the workout habits that you should have:

WORKOUT HABIT 1: Build Right Mindset

To develop good workout habits that are sure to enable you to achieve your goal of losing belly fat, you have to first prepare yourself mentally. The process of regaining shape starts with your mind, and this is half the work. Once you have overcome any mental obstacles, you will be able to have a flat tummy and luckily you might see your abs for the first time in your life. You should commit yourself to the workout sessions otherwise you will end up with negative. Commitment is not about money value; rather it is about being focused and consistent in your workouts. Most people fail in losing belly fat because they quit early because they lose sight of what is really important. They come up with excuses such as they do not have the time to keep up with the workouts or they lack the money to hit the gym.   Some actually do not even see the gym entrance because of their excuses. Others quit after taking a break from working out and end up never making back to the gym and quitting. Others are very weak mentally and can't handle the muscle pain and soreness that come with the workout sessions and end up quitting. This is a backwards mentality and these people have settled for less instead of making the best of their lives and time. Such people have poor willpower and lack the guts to withstand the challenges in working out and getting rid of the belly fat. Losing belly fat and getting in shape guarantees a healthy life free of various lifestyle and health complications.

To develop and maintain effective workout habits you have to develop a positive mindset about working out. You have to be motivated to work out and maintain a consistent schedule. One can stay motivated intrinsically and extrinsically when working on losing the belly fat. This is one of the main reason most gyms contain motivation quotes from successful athletes to keep you going. For example, you can find a photo of Dwayne Johnson with a mention of one of his quotes. This motivates those working out to keep on going if they want to be successful as Dwayne Johnson. This is a form of extrinsic motivation. Your peers can also be a source of extrinsic motivation; you can choose to have friends who have the same goal as you that is losing the belly fat. You can also use music with high energy when exercising. Music pushes your body to move beyond its limits and keep the body excited and the adrenaline flowing.

Extrinsic motivation may be effective it is only for a short time. It can be less effective for people prone to laziness and procrastination which is partly to blame for the belly fat. To go the whole mile in belly fat loss, intrinsic motivation is pivotal. Intrinsic motivation refers to the willpower and how strong it can be to keep you going in your workouts. Intrinsic motivation results from your core values and principles that you believe in. It is what makes you wake up from the bed and quickly get out and go on your morning jogs. It is this motivation that makes you endure the pain when doing your reps when working out. For you to develop this motivation, you have to know the main reason you are working out. Your main motive should be to lose the belly fat. You should also look at the benefits that come with getting rid of the belly fat. The benefits can include having an attractive look, reducing cholesterol levels in the body, getting the job you always wanted.

WORKOUT HABIT 2: Set Work Out Goals

Based on your intrinsic motivation, you should be able to develop your workout goals. They will provide you with a blueprint to follow when you are working out. Your workout goals should be measurable and achievable. For example, you don't expect to lose all the belly fat within a week. Your goal for losing the belly fat may be to improve your work delivery or help you look attractive.

WORKOUT HABIT 3: Make Commitment

The people you see that are always in shape and you have never seen them with a protruding tummy, work on themselves to maintain that look. The following are very effective workout habits that ensure they always have a flat belly or have their abs showing always. There is no magical wand involved but discipline and commitment in sticking to their workout habits. As you begin working out to lose the belly fat, you will need all the motivation you can master to keep going. If you consistently keep doing the same workout exercises at the same time of the day Week-in and week-out, you will eventually develop workout habits. When the workout sessions grow to habits, they become part of your life. Actually, you don't require any persuasions to carry them out. You just do them like any ordinary daily activity. If you develop workout habits not only will you lose the belly fat but be also to maintain the flat or toned belly and stay in shape.

WORKOUT HABIT 4: Start Workout The Right Way

Starting the right way helps you determine the risks you might encounter and helps you sets the targets and goals you wish to achieve during working out. You should start your workout plan the right way, by considering the following:

1) Consult A Physician

It is important that you consult a doctor before embarking on a workout plan. This helps you to know if your body can withstand the exercises. There have been cases of people dying in gyms because of various body conditions that could have been identified by a physician. Don't overlook this option and go on to exercising without seeing a physician, you may be diabetic which may cause complications when working out.

2) Take Your Baseline Measurements

After coming up with your goals, you have to take measurements of your body dimensions. This will help you monitor your progress as you work out. You have to measure your weight especially to help you know how fast you are losing unwanted body fat. Keeping a record of your weight fluctuations will motivate you to keep going with the workout session and you will lose all the belly fat in due time.

3) Develop Workout Habits

The people you see that are always in shape and you have never seen them with a protruding tummy, work on themselves to maintain that look. The following are very effective workout habits that ensure they always have a flat belly or have their abs showing always. There is no magical wand involved but discipline and commitment in sticking to their workout habits. As you begin working out to lose the belly fat, you will need all the motivation you can master to keep going. If you consistently keep doing the same workout exercises at the same time of the day Week-in and week-out, you will eventually develop workout habits. When the workout sessions grow to habits, they become part of your life. Actually, you don't require any persuasions to carry them out. You just do them like any ordinary daily activity. If you develop workout habits not only will you lose the belly fat but be also to maintain the flat or toned belly and stay in shape.

WORKOUT HABIT 5: Take It One Step At A Time

When you start working out, do not be in a hurry. Do every set of exercise in an orderly fashion. In case you are doing 10 sets of pushups, don't give up on the seventh rather push through to the tenth. Then take at least 30 seconds to rest before doing another set of a different exercise such as sit ups. You should have a minimum of 4 sets of different exercises to carry out. When you have done all sets, you can choose to restart in an orderly manner, from the set you started with to the one you ended with.

WORKOUT HABIT 6: Maintain Perseverance

It is going to be hard for you when you start exercising. You will feel your heart beating too fast and feel like you are about to get a heart attack. You may have muscle aches from all the exercising and being a first time in a long time to work out. However, as you continue to work out your body will adapt to the exercises and you will be at ease with the exercises. The burning sensation on your body is a good sign of calories burning and you are starting to lose the excess calories. Never quit, just keep going and when you are tired and out of breath, take a rest.

WORKOUT HABIT 7: Get to The Fatigued Point

In exercising, fatigue is a marker of good exercising. To make progress in losing the belly fat, you have to get to the fatigued point. At the point of fatigue, all your body areas including the belly area have been targeted by the exercises and you are going to lose a a considerable amount of calories. Always strive to exercise until you reach this point to ensure effective burning of belly fat.

WORKOUT HABIT 8: Work on Core Toning

The core of your body is made up of sets of muscles that include the rectus adominus, a large muscle running from the ribcage to the pelvis; and the oblique muscles, which are located on either side. The belly fat covers the core of your body thus you should exercise your core muscles which help in losing the belly fat. So, you should work on toning your core so that you effectively burn a considerable belly fat amount with every workout.

WORKOUT HABIT 9: Love Plank Moves

The plank exercises are effective in helping burn belly fat. They tend to place your body in a different and challenging position than crunches can. A good example of plank moves is the side plank where you have to support your whole body with only two contact surfaces with the floor. The exercise may seem easy to perform but has proved quite challenging irrespective of fitness level. The following are steps in executing the side plank:

1) Lie on one side placing your elbow directly under your shoulder.

2) Maintain the position in (1) raise and place your other arm on your hip.

3) With the arm on your hip raise your bottom hip off the ground by pulling in your abdominals.

4) Hold this plank position for a minimum 30 seconds before lowering back down.

After you have done a set, you should switch to the other side and repeat the steps. In case you have difficulties in getting your bottom hip off the ground you can modify by placing your arm in front of you instead of on your hip to provide extra support. The plank moves are very effective and highly recommended when losing the belly fat. When combined with cardio exercises, they can help lose the belly fat and strengthen the core giving you a lean and healthy body.

WORKOUT HABIT 10: Do Cardio Target Toning

Cardio target toning involves doing cardio exercises in losing belly fat. To effectively lose the belly fat, cardio exercises have to be incorporated. Cardio exercises build your body stamina and help you endure more intense workouts with time. The cardio exercises can be classified into high intensity and less intense. High intensity and endurance training help you lose belly fat at a faster rate. Examples of high-intensity cardio exercises include mountain climbing, jumping jacks and high knees. Less intense cardio exercises include walking, jogging, running, swimming and biking. You can take advantage of the machines provided in the gym such as the stationary bikes and treadmills for your cardio exercises.

WORKOUT HABIT 11: Perform The Crunches

The Crunch is an outstanding exercise for a fat-free belly. It's not difficult to do than the regular sit-up, and it is still just as effective in also strengthening your abs. The ways and means to carry out the crunches are by:

a) The Elbow To Knee Crunches

This is one of the best workouts for a flat belly. Before you learn how to do this exercise, know that you should not perform it if you have a lower back problem or neck problems.

The ways and means to execute this exercise are:

1) Lay on your back and then bring your knees up towards your chest.

2) Put your hands behind your head with your elbows extended out. Then lift your head and shoulders off of the floor. Do not lift with your neck, but lift with the abs.

3) Next step is to extend one leg out as you twist your body so that your elbow comes in toward the opposite knee that is bent.

4) As you twist in the opposite direction pulling your extended leg in towards you while at the same time extending your other leg you should inhale.

5) Try to keep your lower back pressed into the floor, and keep your abs contracted so that you stay balanced.

b) Bicycle Crunches

Bicycle crunches are more effective in that they work more than one group of muscles at the same time. Try this exercise out by:

1) First lying on your back

2) Place your hands behind your head

3) Bring your knees to a 90-degree angle.

4) Twist your upper body to the left, bringing your right elbow to your left knee. Do not pull your neck when doing this manoeuvre.

5) At the same time, extend your right leg above the ground. Return to the centre and repeat on the other side, going at a pace that's comfortable for you.

WORKOUT HABIT 12: Set Up A Dedicated Time For Workout

When creating a workout plan for belly fat loss, you should always consider the time you have set for each set of exercises. For example, you can choose to work out for a duration of an hour with a set of 5 different exercises involved. This requires you to divide the hour in accordance with the level of intensity of each workout exercise. You can choose to spend more time on an exercise that is hard for you and it may take time for you to build up to the intensity it requires.

WORKOUT HABIT 13: Keep Up Your FLAT BELLY WORKOUT ROUTINE

Keeping up with your workout routine will be very vital in getting rid of the belly fat. Workout routines differ from one person to another, below is an example of a workout routine that has proved very effective in getting rid of belly fat. You should not be surprised by the intensity of the exercises rather start slow and build in them. Losing the belly fat completely will not happen in a day, so you have to keep on exercising with your workout plan until the belly fat has disappeared completely.

1) 50 jumping jacks

2) 40 crunches

3) 40 squats

4) 40 leg lifts

5) 30 jumping jacks

6) 20 bicycle crunches

7) 20 squats

8) 30 leg lifts

9) 10 minute cardio exercise

When working out to lose the belly fat, start slow and increase the intensity and length of the exercises over time. With time you will feel a burning sensation that might be intense from time to time. This burning sensation is as a result of your abdominal muscles burning calories as you workout. When you are losing the belly fat, use exercises that target the core. You should also use cardio exercises as much as possible. Avoid trying weightlifting to lose the belly fat. Weightlifting is ineffective in losing belly fat and you should use body weight exercises and cardio exercises to target the belly area and get the fat around the area burning and reducing.

WORKOUT HABIT 14: Mix Different Exercises

You should also mix your exercises to effectively lose the belly fat. You can't lose belly fat completely if you only resort to one or two exercises. Choose exercises that target the core and effectively work it out ensuring that you keep on losing the belly fat and getting in shape. You can also effectively lose the belly fat by increasing the reps in your exercises. The more reps you add to your exercises, the more calories you are burning which will greatly help in getting rid of the belly fat.

WORKOUT HABIT 15: Add More Reps

Keep adding more reps and you will soon realize that your belly fat is reducing and your core is becoming stronger at the same time. Always remember to start slow and build upon the intensity of the exercises with time. It is more convenient to get in more reps rather than wear yourself out quickly with an exercise that is too intense. Our bodies are different and some people lose their belly fat faster than others. Stick to your workout plan and work on losing the belly fat every day and you will soon get the results you are looking for.

PART 3:
LIFESTYLE HABITS

The lifestyle habits you choose also have a bigger role to play in you having a big belly. Most people especially those well off have the idea that having a belly is a normal thing for people in their stature. They associate having a belly with their wealth. This is a backwards notion as a flat tummy guarantees you a more healthy life than having a big belly. Do not ignore the belly because you think your life is fun enough and you do not have to stress about your appearance. Your body is a very delicate object than you think, if you don't take care of it, it will break into pieces. A belly may be a source of many health complications because of the fat concentrated in the belly area and your unwillingness to get rid of it. The best lifestyle to live is that geared towards taking care of your well-being and making your life free of drama and diseases. All around, there are different cases of people succumbing to lifestyle diseases such as diabetes and certain cancers. This can be avoided if you shape your life to be something that makes you stronger with time rather than weakens you with time. The following are what you should include in your life to ensure that you are able to lose the belly fat and maintain the lean body:

LIFESTYLE HABIT 1: Get Adequate Sleep

Research shows that sleep is a very important ingredient in having a healthy body. Most people have become workaholics, working two jobs daily or working overtime. This does not allow them to have adequate sleep that is essential for the human body metabolism and growth. The human body requires a minimum of 7-8 hours of peaceful sleep daily. You should choose a daily routine where you have to sleep adequately and be able to allow your body to rest. You should train your body to sleep in time to have the adequate time required to sleep and make it in time to wake up in time for your daily activities. Sleep plays a big role in helping you lose fat, as the body is able to break down the excess fats around the abdominal area to provide energy for cell metabolism and muscle growth.

People who adapt to the "early to bed and early to rise" lifestyle are active in life and always energetic to carry out their daily activities. Adequate sleep makes your body feel refreshed and full of energy. The excited state of your body allows your mind to focus on the productive activities rather than concentrating on food and overeating, hence the belly fat will not fade. You should also avoid sleeping during the day as much as you can, as this makes you feel lethargic and may encourage you to think about food which in turn makes you eat a lot in one day. Make exceptions in days when you have had a very busy and exhausting work time.

LIFESTYLE HABIT 2: Have Emotional Freedom

Belly fat is also encouraged by a lifestyle filled with emotional stress. This is because emotional stress increases the levels of the cortisol stress hormone, which is scientifically associated with belly fat accumulation. Thus, even though stress is inevitable in our day to day lives, you should adopt a lifestyle that helps you alleviate it. Stress without exercising can result in the fast accumulation of belly fat. In case, you are stressed you should hit the gym and blow off some steam by exercising. Exercising helps you to keep your body active and keep your stress levels low.

Never let the pressures of life weigh you down and result to you having an unattractive body cupped by a big belly. Don't allow yourself to fall deep into alcohol and drug abuse, which also increase the cortisol stress hormone. The best way to go is to find healthy ways to reduce the stress levels of working out in the gym. This keeps you going in losing belly fat and attaining a healthy and lean body.

LIFESTYLE HABIT 3: Change From A Sedentary Lifestyle To An Active One

Some people lives lack fun and is quite sad and lethargic. This is not the best lifestyle to live when you want to lose the belly fat. You should learn to make your life active so as to always maintain your body feeling energetic and able to work out. An active lifestyle makes your life worthwhile, relieving you of stress and encouraging you to work hard to lose the belly fat.

You can have an active life by going on vacations when free. This allows you to see the world and learn different cultures. You can also take your family on a picnic, go for a swim, walk or bicycle ride. In your mind, you are just having fun, but in a real sense, you are burning excess calories and hence keep losing the belly fat.

LIFESTYLE HABIT 4: Make A Life Plan And Be Patient

Most things in life go wrong because of failing to plan, so is gaining belly fat. The people you see with fine and athletic bodies free of belly fat are not demigods. They are human like you and all they had to do is lay out a life plan and in it list measures of having a healthy and lean body and adhered to them. So, to have a lifestyle that you know where you are going is an important ingredient in having a flat belly. Have a plan on how you are not only going to lose the belly fat but also have a healthy body. Be patient with your plan as and don't expect immediate results. Trust in the process and with time, you will have a healthy and lean body with a happy life as a bonus.

LIFESTYLE HABIT 5: Follow Your Dreams And Talents

As people grow older, they give up on their talents as they settle in live and take up various responsibility roles. To have a healthy lifestyle free of a belly fat to struggle with do not let go of things you were good at. For example, you were a good soccer player but you ended up becoming a lawyer. You should take time in your weekends to go and watch a soccer match, better still you can join a local soccer team and play some soccer. This keeps you active and you maintain a healthy and fit body. Life is not about giving up and it is important that you always maintain a healthy life by always being physically active on a daily basis. One of these physical activities involves working on your talents.

Working on your talents also distracts you from your unhealthy eating habits enabling you to control your cravings. This, in turn, helps you to shed the belly fat and stay fit and healthy.

LIFESTYLE HABIT 6: Foster Healthy Friendships

Another lifestyle habit that you should embrace is having friends in your corner who encourage you to work out and stay fit. You can't make it alone in life and need others to help and push you on. You should embrace a social lifestyle that enables you to stay happy and healthy at the same time. For example, you should have gym buddies who you go with to work out in the gym. You can have friends who encourage you to avoid certain types of foods that can result in you gaining weight and losing your flat belly. In short, you should have friends who share the same fitness goals as you.

LIFESTYLE HABIT 7: Undergo Medical Check Up

Build a culture of going to visit the doctor for a medical checkup even when you are not ill. This is related to having a healthy and belly in that the doctor is able to advise you on what workouts are effective in maintaining a lean body. The doctor is also able to determine if you are missing out on any essential nutrients in your dieting.

LIFESTYLE HABIT 8: Practice Meditation

Meditating supplements the efforts you are putting in losing the belly fat. You can do all the exercises imaginable, adopt all the healthy eating habits and still have belly fat. The aim of meditating is to relax and clear the mind, thus reducing stress levels. This lowers the cortisol stress hormone levels. Meditation also helps you have an adequate and improved sleep, lowers blood sugar and boosts both the body metabolism and immunity. These factors are vital in helping you lose the belly fat. It is therefore important that you include meditation sessions in your daily routines. It will prove effective in losing the belly fat.

CONCLUSION

After reading this book, you are now well equipped with the knowledge of how to lose that belly fat that has been causing you distress. You have realized that the problem is you and all it takes is you changing your daily unhealthy habits and embracing new and healthier ones. Do not lose your self-confidence because your belly fat is making you lose friends and maybe making you ineffective in your job. You have to believe that you can get rid of the belly fat and prove those who look down on you because of the belly fat wrong. A flat belly or chiselled abdomen guarantees a healthy life free from complications like heart disease and cholesterol. A flat belly is a sign of good healthy and makes you look attractive and hence a good social life.

You should know that losing belly fat is not hard, but maintaining that flat belly is the hardest part. After losing the belly fat, do not fall off the wagon and go back to the habits that resulted to the belly fat in the first place. You just have to adapt a plan and lifestyle that ensures that you do not get the belly fat back again. This book has provided insights on how you should ensure that the belly fat is gone for good. Stick to these insights and you will live a good life where you do not have to worry about belly fat. Remember to be committed and have a positive mind when you are working to lose the belly fat.

www.ingramcontent.com/pod-product-compliance
Lightning Source LLC
Chambersburg PA
CBHW071114280526
45787CB00003B/1040